Talantbek Abdullaevich Batyraliev
Mederbek Adyshevich Ismailov
Bolot Aripovich Abilov

Implementation of public-private partnership in the healthcare system

Talantbek Abdullaevich Batyraliev
Mederbek Adyshevich Ismailov
Bolot Aripovich Abilov

Implementation of public-private partnership in the healthcare system

Challenges and prospects

ScienciaScripts

Cover image: www.ingimage.com

This book is a translation from the original published under ISBN 978-620-2-05744-8.

Publisher:
Sciencia Scripts
is a trademark of
Dodo Books Indian Ocean Ltd. and OmniScriptum S.R.L publishing group

120 High Road, East Finchley, London, N2 9ED, United Kingdom
Str. Armeneasca 28/1, office 1, Chisinau MD-2012, Republic of Moldova, Europe
Printed at: see last page
ISBN: 978-620-7-79522-2

Table of Contents

Chapter 1

Introduction. Relevance.

As it is known, the problems of public-private partnership (hereinafter - PPP) development in the modern development of many countries of the world and its role in the formation of the innovation component of the economic system and improving the competitiveness of the latter are constantly in the centre of attention of many government and public figures, as well as scientists and practitioners [2, 5, 13, 18].

In most post-Soviet countries, including the Kyrgyz Republic (hereinafter - KR), the formation and development of a market economy and new economic relations is proceeding at different rates.

The economies of the Commonwealth of Independent States (CIS) are striving for greater integration with Western democracies, with a pressing need for structural change and closer co-operation between the state and the private sector.

This interaction is formed on such a platform as PPP, which has recently acquired a very significant role, acting in the eyes of the world community as one of the most effective and promising structural components for the successful implementation of various investment projects, including in the field of health care. The legitimate interest in this interaction on the part of public structures and the private sector can be explained primarily by the fact that in many countries PPP allows to effectively solve major social and economic problems by combining the resources of public and private investors [12, 17].

At the same time, it is believed that the improvement of PPP mechanisms and the formation of new structures in the economic system contributes to attracting direct investments into the economy, and the improvement of the quality of services provided to the population will contribute to the growth of competitiveness of local economic systems.

All this will ultimately have a favourable impact on the process of formation of the innovation economy.

In the conditions of functioning of progressive partnership relations, new effective management methods and financing models based on significant changes in the relations between forms of ownership appear [1, 3, 9].

Thus, the formation of innovative relations is closely correlated with changes in the institutional environment.

The complexity of issues related to the development of PPPs in the conditions accompanied by the economic and financial crisis puts before economic science the task to conduct a thorough analysis, monitoring and evaluation of the current situation. The high practical significance of analysing and evaluating new structures functioning on the basis of PPPs determined the relevance of this monograph.

The scientific foundations for the study of PPP theory in the world economic literature are presented in the works of such venerable scientists as Adam Smith, Bow P., Johansson F., Karloff B., Keins J., Koase R., Mankiw G., David Ricardo, William F. Sharpe and others. Sharpe et al. The works of these authors had a direct impact on the formation and development of the theory of interaction between the state and private business.

The study of the impact of PPP on the formation of a market economy, as well as its modernisation in modern conditions in the CIS territory, has its roots in the early 1990s of the twentieth century. This fact has a close relationship with the collapse of the planned Soviet economy.

At the same time, despite the great attention to the problems of PPP formation and development, many issues remain insufficiently studied. In particular, there is no complete clarity in the settlement of ownership rights between the state and the private sector of the economy.

There are still issues related to clarifying the role and place of institutional transformations as one of the most important factors in rationalising the interaction between the state and business. The problems and prospects of PPP improvement in the innovation sphere require further study [4, 10].

The next steps for further scientific support for the development of PPP principles are the development of theoretical, methodological and scientific and practical recommendations to identify promising forms of PPP development in the conditions of economic modernisation, activation of innovation relations at the current stage of society development.

In this regard, it is essential:

- clarify the essence of PPPs as an economic category , through

  systematise concepts and theories, and provide a critical assessment of structural and procedural approaches to its definition;

- analyse models and forms of interaction (partnership) between the state and business in the modern economy and identify their advantages and disadvantages;
- identify ways to optimise ownership rights between the state and the private sector of the economy;
- identify the role and place of institutional transformations in rationalising the interaction between the state and business in the process of modernisation and diversification of the economy;
- to identify the peculiarities of PPP improvement in the innovation sphere.

These areas of activity require the use of special research methods. These include, first of all: methods of systematic and complex approach to the analysis of economic phenomena: analysis and synthesis, method of scientific abstraction, economic and statistical method, as well as the method of expert assessments.

On the other hand, with regard to the social component of the sphere of economic activity of the society, it should be understood that the health of the nation is a strategic resource of the country, the basis for the formation of human capital and the foundation for the development of the national economy.

In turn, the state of the national economy depends on the use of innovative models of development of various spheres and industries.

The healthcare sector is no exception, the innovative development of which should be aimed at further reforming, developing and implementing innovations in medicine, identifying new sources of financing, and forming modern healthcare management tools.

The experience of many developed countries shows that the implementation of PPP system takes a leading position in socio-economic development. To ensure the development of the social sphere, including health care, it is necessary to attract additional capital, which should come from the implementation of forms of cooperation between the state and private business [5].

Chapter 2

Forms of partnership in world practice.

In the world practice, as is known, there are two forms of partnership: institutional and contractual. The institutional form involves the creation of joint ventures with the participation of the state and business [1, 15, 16].

In healthcare, this form can be implemented in the following ways.

- Creation of a new medical organisation with joint participation of the state and business.
- Establishment of a non-profit organisation in the healthcare sector
- Establishment of a management company for implementation and management of healthcare projects
- Transfer to a private company of a share of a state medical organisation (including partial privatisation).

With regard to the latter, an example is the possible transfer of a maternity hospital, which is a structural part of a state-owned health care organisation (hereinafter - HCO). This option does not currently have appropriate legal and regulatory support. Its practical implementation is possible using a contractual form of strategic partnership, which implies the conclusion of a contract for the performance of certain functions in relation to a particular health care facility.

Classification of contractual forms in health care:

Depending on who is the payer of the contracted health care services provided:

- Concession (concession agreement) is a specific form of relations between the state and a private partner, the peculiarity of which lies in the fact that the state (or a municipal entity) in the framework of partnership relations, remaining the full owner of the medical organisation, transfers to the private partner the performance of the functions specified in the agreement for a certain period of time and grants it, for this purpose, the relevant powers necessary to ensure the normal functioning of the object of concession (for the use of the services provided by the concessionaire, the user pays for the services provided by the concessionaire) [2]. The user pays for the services provided by the concessionaire) [2].

- Private Finance Initiative - contracts for public services and works financed by the private sector cover the same elements, but for practical reasons are paid for by the state rather than consumers [1].

Depending on the availability of rights to transfer the subject matter of the contract to the private partner:

- with the right to transfer to a medical organisation;
- without the right to transfer to a medical organisation.

Depending on the functions transferred to the private partner:

- designing a medical organisation
- construction of a medical organisation
- reconstruction of a medical organisation
- maintenance of infrastructure by the medical organisation
- medical organisation management
- funding.

Contractual forms of quasi - PPPs

- a contract for the provision of medical services by private organisations;
- a co-operation agreement;
- a contract for the performance of auxiliary functions of a medical organisation (outsourcing).

Based on the analysis, in accordance with the international classification, it is proposed to use the following basic models of PPP contractual form for the health care system [6].

The application of the models presented below is primarily aimed at solving actual problems in the health care system through the possibility of providing the necessary volume and types of paid medical services. In this case, payment for services is made in stages, taking into account the time period established by the contract. The decision to implement a particular model should be made by the public partner only when there is strong evidence that the private partner has the professional competences to carry out the activities sought.

Basic models of contractual PPPs

Currently, 6 basic models of PPP contractual form in healthcare are distinguished.

Model #1. A private partner undertakes to modernise and reconstruct a state-owned OZ. After the work is completed, it starts to carry out its activities using the infrastructure of the OZ for a specific period of time specified in the PPP Agreement. The specified period of time is determined taking into account the interests of the private partner, which should be sufficient for the investor to recover the funds spent. Works on reconstruction and further maintenance of OZ require significant financial investments. The profitability of a PPP project directly depends on the amount of payments from the state for the work performed. The state partner finds such a model most acceptable for use only when there is a chronic deficit of budget financing. At the same time, modernisation of OZ is aimed at solving current problems in the health care system.

Model 2: The main difference from the first model is the delegated right for the private partner to receive payment for health services from the population.

This model focuses on equity between partners in funding issues.

At the initial stage of modernisation, the private partner finances the modernisation process in full, and later the public partner pays a share of the costs for a contractually agreed period of time.

Services can be provided by the reconstructed EH both for cash and under compulsory or voluntary health insurance programmes. A private partner will be interested in this model if it provides the necessary return for the invested capital and guarantees a profit.

The state pays for services rendered under the compulsory medical insurance system (hereinafter - CMI) and paid medical services. The ratio of MHI and paid services depends on the share of reimbursement by the state of the initial investments in reconstruction.

Under this model, the following variant can be considered, positioned as a private financial initiative and expressed in the fact that the private partner does not participate in the MHI system and provides only paid medical services, paying rent to the state.

Model #3. The use of this model implies the transfer of OZ in trust management to a private partner. The relevance of this model is conditioned by the fact that the state has some OZ designed to solve problems in the field of health care, but with fixed high costs, and the lack of possibility to provide effective management for its management and provision of high quality medical services. The choice of this model by the state may be conditioned by the absence of an investor at the initial stage, but while maintaining the need to solve the problem in a short period of time, as well as by the impossibility of ensuring the operation of the HSS and the provision of medical services without the participation of a private partner.

The private partner will be interested in this model if it provides the required efficiency. Services are provided both under the MHI system and for cash. The state pays for MHI services

In this case, the following option may be considered, where the private partner does not provide health services, but provides infrastructure services to the PPH. This model can be applied to existing health centres that do not need to be reconstructed.

Model No. 4. This model involves the construction (or performance of part of the construction work) of a medical organisation by a private partner in accordance with the state's assignment; upon completion of construction, the medical organisation is transferred to the state partner and handed over to the private partner for a certain period of time for use without the right of ownership. The private partner carries out maintenance work on the infrastructure of the medical organisation, but may not provide medical services. The private partner receives a fee from the state for the service. The state benefits from this model if it does not have sufficient funds to build a medical organisation on its own.

Model No. 5. This model assumes, like model No. 4, that a private partner builds a medical organisation in accordance with the state's assignment; upon completion of construction, the medical organisation is transferred to the state partner. Unlike Model 4, the private partner receives the right to provide medical services and manage the medical organisation. This model is favourable for the private partner if the profit received from the provision of services covers the costs and provides the required level of return on investment, taking into account the risks. The state pays for the provision of paid medical services, and the state pays for the provision of services in the MHI system. The ratio of MHI and paid services largely depends on the share of reimbursement by the state of initial investments in the construction of a medical organisation.

Model #6. This model assumes that the state attracts a private partner only to finance the construction or reconstruction of OZ. The private partner is interested in receiving a return of funds including interest.

For each model, a prerequisite is the establishment of indicators to monitor and control the actions of the private partner.

It has now been shown that the initiation of PPP projects is desirable precisely in those areas where privatisation processes are impossible.

These include: energy sector; roads and railways; gas, water and heat supply; agriculture, as well as social spheres: health care, education and housing and utilities [17].

The choice of the most optimal model of interaction between the state and business largely depends on the depth of scientific study of the project, investment model, its participants and other criteria. In the conditions of economic reforms, such forms as concessions, delegated management, production sharing agreements [15, 16] are getting the greatest development.

PPPs operate on the basis of "splitting of property rights", which are realised through a voluntary exchange of entitlements. The state carries out a partial transfer of certain rights to the property, defined by law and agreement (contract), namely: the right to income, the right to management, the right to control the use of assets, the right to change the capital value of the objects of agreements and the right to assign certain ownership rights to other persons.

However, this is possible if two conditions are met:

- the owner's consent to the relevant disposal operation (sale, exchange, donation, etc.);
- to use the funds received strictly for their intended purpose.

Based on the use of a systematic approach, it was determined that the most important factor in improving the efficiency of PPP functioning is a civilised institutional environment. It forms the constraints on the activities of economic entities of public-private partnership, and the basis of the institutional environment is formed, in turn, by property institutions. They have a direct impact on economic growth, allocation of resources, income distribution, employment and real income.

They are directly related to actions that influence the correlation between personal and public interest, decision-making procedures.

The main areas of activity to improve PPPs in various spheres of the economy are such as:

- development of legislative and regulatory legal acts and organisational mechanisms regulating PPP development from the position of ensuring a balance of interests of all its participants;
- provision of guarantees for business loans for the introduction of knowledge-intensive technologies;
- Creating favourable framework conditions to ensure that

  Interaction between the public and private sectors of the economy through mandatory involvement of sectoral business associations in the formation, co-financing and evaluation of performance

  fulfilment of public-private contracts;
- subsidising a certain part of business expenses on scientific research and transferring the created scientific and technical products to repay the debts of business structures to the state;
- practical use of the results of scientific research on the basis of implementation of innovation and investment projects;
- expansion of mechanisms for the provision of budget guarantees for non-commercial risks to ensure the inflow of investments for the development of innovative structures.

The next problem for the successful implementation of PPP principles is the lack of coordination between agencies, the length of coordination of various aspects of the project, the lack of real responsibility in government structures are perceived by the business community as more significant shortcomings than the failure of the state to fulfil its obligations under the contract or the desire for excessive control over the private partner.

In the CIS countries, there are still significant gaps in the legislation governing economic activities on state-owned properties with private sector participation.

The institutions of public law and property, as well as others, within which the whole system of partnership relations between the state and the private sector in developed countries functions, are absent. Relations between business and the state are still difficult to call trust-based. Partnerships can fit into various legal frameworks that create prerequisites and basis for business participation in the management of state property.

Two ways of organising partnerships from a legal perspective can be distinguished.

The first option is the evolutionary ingrowth of PPPs into the existing legal system of directly applicable and indirect legislation.

In aggregate, a sufficiently extensive system of legal provisions for the normal functioning of partnership relations is formed.

It includes laws providing various regimes for the use of state property and currency exchange, civil and tax codes, contract law, laws regulating the use of state property and currency exchange, and laws regulating the use of foreign exchange.

investment investments, etc.

The second option involves the development of a new, stable institutional and legal framework. In this case, partnerships are formed within the framework of special legislative acts, and the activities of partners are regulated by dozens of annexes designed to make up for the absence of contract law.

Despite the proven advantages and undoubted successes in the development of PPPs in foreign countries, the use of this mechanism in the CIS countries remains an alternative, rather than the main way of solving problems in the field of public goods provision.

The fact is that PPP institutional systems cannot be exported like manufactured goods, but are created over decades [2].

One of the important reasons constraining the development of the PPP system in the CIS is the lack of a unified management system. The most important factor for the successful development of PPPs is the coordination of actions of government agencies in the development and implementation of projects, the lack of which is one of the main problems. Each ministry tries to supervise its own projects and create its own programmes. All this may lead to deterioration of the competitive environment in the region.

On the other hand, the complexity of the projects to be implemented is likely to result in high transaction costs. The practice of partnership, especially at the initial stage - searching for partners and project development - is associated with significant costs (costs of tenders, expertise, legal and consulting services). In addition, the use of such a form as project financing, due to the significant risks involved, can be fraught with the payment of higher interest on loans and commissions to various third-party corporations and organisations involved in the process.

Increased transaction costs may be accompanied by increased administrative costs of reorganising the apparatus at all levels affected by PPPs. However, these costs are usually offset by the benefits of private financing.

An important point is that it is impossible to adjust the terms of the agreement in case of unfavourable for the state changes in external conditions (financial, environmental or other) in the course of the agreement [11].

We cannot ignore such aspect as insufficient information provision on priority areas for the implementation of investment projects, which negatively affects investment activity. Therefore, it is necessary to conduct awareness-raising campaigns about PPP in mass media.

In addition, the authorities at the local level are often unable to assess the potential of PPPs, as well as to put it on a practical basis, primarily due to the lack of knowledge about PPPs and the lack of specialists with experience in the implementation of partnership projects [6]. It follows that a new system of training and professional development of officials on PPP problems, as well as training and graduation of young specialists in this field is required. For this purpose, it is necessary, on the one hand, to strengthen the relevant motivation, and, on the other hand, to fix all this in the relevant legislative acts.

Chapter 3

Problems of interaction between public and private health care.

Insufficiently high economic efficiency of functioning of state EI (due to the specifics of this organisational-legal form of ownership) in the conditions of market relations, limited public resources and other factors inevitably raise the question of finding ways to attract private investment in the sector, acceptable forms of relations between budgetary EI and private organisations, borrowing the experience of commercial structures to improve the activities of budgetary institutions.

As the non-state health care sector develops and investments in private health care increase, the problem of interaction between the state and private medical organisations becomes more and more urgent.

Improvement of the economic situation of the country, growth of the size of budgets leads to the fact that private medical organisations are increasingly interested in public resources in the form of budgets of all levels and funds of compulsory health insurance. Therefore, it is private health care that most often raises the question of interaction between public and private health care.

The development of private health care and the interaction between the public and private sector are quite complex problems, combining both positive and negative aspects.

In addition to the traditional benefits of business development (increased employment, tax revenues, etc.), the positive aspects of for-profit healthcare development include:

- attraction of additional financial resources (funds of the population and enterprises) to health care;
- public health savings, which are achieved by the affluent part of the population seeking commercial services. This improves the delivery of health care to the rest of the population;
- the emergence of an opportunity for medical personnel of public health care institutions to earn additional income by providing paid services or working part-time in private medical organisations (which is a common practice worldwide).

All this indicates the need to support private healthcare. Especially since the task of the state is to take care not only of state and municipal budgetary medical institutions, but also of private healthcare.

For example, Article 47 of the Constitution of the Kyrgyz Republic states that: "The state shall create conditions for medical care for everyone and shall take measures to develop the state, municipal and private health care sectors" [8] [8].

At the same time, one cannot ignore the fact that the development of private health care is closely dependent on the state of public health care. Unsatisfied demand for free medical care inevitably gives rise to demand for paid services.

However, the forms in which these paid services are provided may vary:

- shadow payment for services in budgetary institutions (the most undesirable form);
- official development of paid medical services in budgetary institutions;
- provision of services in OZ with private ownership.

It should be noted that according to foreign and domestic experts, the development of private health care is more preferable than the provision of paid services in public institutions. The combination of free medical care and entrepreneurial activity (provision of paid services) in state (municipal) health care organisations does not allow for effective control over the targeted use of budgetary funds and mandatory health insurance (hereinafter - MHI) funds.

Such a combination inevitably gives rise to prerequisites for either financial violations or violations of citizens' rights to free medical care (although, of course, these prerequisites are not always realised in practice).

In the long term, the provision of paid medical services (at least for cash payment) should be discontinued in budget-funded institutions. However, this presupposes certain conditions:

- a well-developed network of private healthcare organisations;
- high solvent demand for medical services on the part of the population;
- sufficient level of financing of budgetary institutions.

Unfortunately, all this is not yet in place, and paid medical services in budget-funded institutions will continue to exist for quite a long time. Therefore, an effective mechanism of control over the development of paid medical services should be developed.

Emphasis should be placed on the development of paid services in specially designated departments, on services and services provided for non-cash payment (to enterprises and organisations, and primarily within the framework of voluntary health insurance).

It should be noted that the influence of the state on the market of commercial medical services is contradictory. The state is able to influence not only the situation in public health care, but also, through this, the price level in the commercial sector: the more accessible and qualitative free medical services are, the lower the demand and prices for paid medical services, and vice versa. Therefore, there is an uneven distribution of types of health services between the markets for paid and free services. In turn, this leads to price disproportionality, when, on the one hand, high prices for commercial services are caused by the impossibility or difficulty of obtaining some services for free (service services, dental services using the latest filling materials, etc.), and on the other hand, relatively low prices for other services are associated with a much greater possibility of obtaining these services for free (types of services included in the MHI programme or financed from the budget).

It should be borne in mind that violation of the procedure for provision of paid medical services in budgetary institutions causes financial damage not only to the population and the budget, but also to private healthcare (due to dumping prices, etc.). State (municipal) health care organisations find themselves in better competitive conditions compared to private organisations not only in case of explicit or implicit financial violations. These advantages are embedded in the differences in the costs of providing medical care: budgetary institutions usually use buildings, facilities free of charge (do not pay rent) and expensive medical equipment, and do not reimburse a number of other costs when providing paid services.

Private EHs are deprived of this opportunity, which objectively forces them to have high prices for similar types of medical services, to focus on scarce, service or high-margin services.

The problem of interaction between public and private health care can be divided into two parts:

1. Interaction of private clinics directly with state and municipal authorities.
2. Interaction of private clinics with budgetary (state and municipal) health care organisations.

Interaction of private clinics directly with state and municipal authorities

When considering the issues of interaction between the state and private healthcare, one cannot leave aside the problem of PPPs. If we talk about the classical understanding of PPP, the main meaning for the state is to attract private investment in the public health sector; to save budgetary funds required for repair and maintenance of neglected health care buildings, which is ensured through the implementation of investment projects.

The main forms of PPPs in the healthcare system at the present stage are the following:

- Establishment (construction) of new private medical centres with government assistance in terms of infrastructure etc..;
- transfer of geographically favourably located buildings of medical institutions to the investor on the terms of construction of new buildings for these medical institutions in other locations;
- renovation of buildings to relocate health care facilities there from other buildings attractive to private investors;
- reorganisation of state medical institutions into joint stock companies with 100% state capital and possible subsequent establishment of a joint public-private enterprise with the participation of a private investor.

As for investment-attractive activities for the private sector (including foreign capital), these may be the following areas:

- remedial treatment;
- high-tech medical care;
- haemodialysis;
- diagnostic service;
- obstetrics;

- technical and economic maintenance of OZ (outsourcing).

With regard to the change of the organisational-legal form of EH, it should be said that despite the existence of such a theoretical possibility, examples of such practice are sporadic.

For example, Russia is currently in the process of reforming a number of state (self-financing) EI into joint-stock companies with one hundred per cent state capital [18].

If we go beyond the classical understanding of PPP, the interaction between the state and private business in healthcare is expressed, among other things, in the direct participation of private medical organisations in the provision of free medical care to the population.

The main forms of such participation are:

- involvement of private medical organisations in the implementation of the territorial MHI programme;
- provision of free-of-charge assistance to the population within the framework of the state (municipal) order.

Theoretically, the most appropriate form of participation of private clinics in free medical care of residents is their integration into the system of compulsory medical insurance. The current legislation allows for this.

Nevertheless, private clinics are very poorly represented in the MHI system. The share of private clinics in the total number of medical organisations operating in the MHI system is low, as well as the share of private medical organisations (out of the total number) providing free medical care under the MHI programme.

This is due, firstly, to the fact that non-state medical organisations most often consider work in the MHI system as an inefficient line of their activities (since only five main items of expenditure are usually reimbursed at the expense of MHI funds and the costs of maintaining buildings, purchasing and operating equipment, etc. are not reimbursed). In part, this problem could be solved within the framework of a pilot project on single-channel financing. However, even in this case private clinics are not fully reimbursed for their costs.

The second problem is that it is very difficult for non-state medical organisations to get an opportunity to work in the MHI system - the state usually gives priority to maintaining budget (even if inefficient) medical institutions rather than sharing limited MHI funds with commercial organisations.

Nevertheless, there is experience of such work of private medical organisations in the MHI system.

Thus, private in-patient clinics such as: ophthalmological centre for eye microsurgery and cardiology centres operate in the Kyrgyz MHI system.

The practice of increasing the participation of private medical organisations in the MHI system needs to be developed, including through more equitable tariffs in the MHI system that take into account the types of costs directly financed by the state for budgetary institutions (related to the maintenance of buildings and facilities).

At the same time, it should be noted that not always the principle of MHI, according to which MHI funds should follow the patients, including private clinics, and patients in private clinics would pay only the difference between the full cost of services in these clinics and the tariffs in the MHI system, is recognised as fair [4, 18].

It should be remembered that the MHI is an imperfect, but still an insurance system, which implies a high degree of social solidarity. In addition, at the expense of MHI, medical care must be provided free of charge to citizens. This means that any citizen, including those who do not want to pay extra for their treatment, should receive free medical care in private medical organisations operating within the MHI system.

Kyrgyzstan is ready to include in the MHI system any private clinic that has a contract for the provision of free medical care under the MHI with an insurance organisation. But the obligation to control the provision of free medical care in this case rests with the insurance organisation itself, which should think carefully before entering into such contracts with private clinics.

In most cases, the participation of private organisations in the MHI system is an attempt to more fully utilise the capacity of their clinics, where, along with free care, paid services not included in the state guarantee programme will be provided.

Another form of participation of private clinics in the provision of free medical care to the population is the state order for medical services. There are also many problems when using the state order, because state or municipal institutions receive budget funds directly from the budget, without a tender, and when conducting competitive procedures, they have a great advantage in terms of the prices offered, as they do not include a number of items in their costs.

Nevertheless, there are a number of examples of a methodologically correct approach to this problem. For example, if the state's capacity to provide the necessary volume of haemodialysis procedures was insufficient, a tender was held to attract private structures, with the inclusion in the price of amortisation, utilities and other costs, which for budgetary institutions were covered directly from the budget.

Interaction of private medical organisations with budgetary institutions

Such interaction can pursue various goals. A review of the practice of relations between state (municipal) and private medical organisations allows us to present a certain classification of these relations:

1. Assistance to budgetary institutions in organising their provision (both free and paid) of medical care.

Let us first consider the problems of providing medical care free of charge to the population with the involvement of private clinics.

First of all, we are talking about the purchase of certain types of services from private organisations by budget institutions. This primarily concerns diagnostic services.

Thus, the issue of using private laboratories as a centralised laboratory financed by the MLA is currently under consideration in the KR.

Among the main reasons that suggest such involvement of private clinics in the promotion of free health care are the following:

- Inability to provide certain types of medical care by budget-funded OBs due to their lack of equipment, necessary personnel, etc. First of all, this applies to small health centres, territorially remote structural subdivisions of medical institutions;
- The economic inexpediency of organising the provision of some types of care (usually diagnostic) by budget institutions, when it is more profitable to purchase certain types of services from private organisations (e.g. services for which the need is low) when these types of care are available from private clinics.

- There are much more opportunities for cooperation between budgetary and private medical organisations when budgetary institutions provide paid medical services. The following possible objectives of co-operation can be indicated:

- Attracting additional commercial patients to budget institutions. For example, working under contracts with private firms that refer patients for treatment to the budget institution. There can be quite a lot of options for co-operation here. Private firms can refer to budget institutions those patients who need specialised care that is not available in private medical institutions; provide information support for the activities of the budget institution; play the role of simple intermediaries, etc.

- Sale of certain types of medical services to private clinics. In this case, it is not the patient but the private medical organisation that buys from the budget institution and pays for services that it cannot provide itself. As a rule, the patient of the private organisation does not have contacts with the budgetary institution (for example, when providing laboratory diagnostics services, etc.), or these contacts do not concern the financial side (the patient, receiving a service, does not pay anything to the budgetary institution, and the invoice is issued to the private firm that referred the patient to the budgetary OIH).

- Provision of additional services or services to provide more comfortable conditions to patients of budget-funded OIH by private organisations. In this case, a budget-funded institution may refuse to provide paid services in this form on its own.

- Providing budgetary institutions with information, reference, analytical, marketing and other services related to the development of entrepreneurial activities.

2. Utilisation of temporarily free capacities of budget institutions.

Temporarily free capacities (premises, equipment) of budget-funded institutions can be provided for use to private medical organisations. It is more advantageous for the state EI that in case of granting premises for use to private firms, it is the organisations carrying out medical activities that act as users. This is due to the fact that in addition to income from the use of property, a budgetary institution, as a rule, gets an opportunity to sell a certain volume of services to a private medical organisation (or its patients) on a paid basis.

It should be noted that temporarily free capacities of budgetary EI are not only empty premises and idle equipment, but also premises and equipment used during one shift and unused during the rest of the day, weekends, etc. Therefore, in a number of cases it is possible for budgetary institutions to provide their facilities to other organisations not on a permanent basis (within an agreed period of time), but only for certain limited periods of time. This could be, for example, the provision of some operating theatres to private clinics in the evening to perform their operations, etc.

3. Attracting additional material resources to the budget institution.

Budget institutions in their turn can also use equipment and premises of private organisations (surplus, temporarily idle, etc.) for entrepreneurial activities.

4. Attracting additional labour resources to the budget institution.

In order to develop entrepreneurial activity, the budgetary institution is interested in expanding both the volume of traditionally provided paid services and in introducing new types of paid services.

It is clear that in a budget-funded institution the same specialists are unlikely to perform the entire scope of prescribed procedures and surgical interventions at an equal quality level, taking into account the existing specialisation of both structural units and doctors themselves. And if in emergency situations surgeons are forced to perform any necessary operations corresponding to the technical capabilities of OZ, regardless of how good the skills of particular doctors are in this area, then in planned and, moreover, paid operations, specialisation is particularly evident.

Developing a certain competence and acquiring the required skills is a complex, time-consuming and expensive process. In most cases, it is most expedient to attract doctors from other institutions, regardless of their organisational and legal form of ownership, on certain conditions. At the same time, attracting doctors from private clinics to work in public OBs acts as a mechanism for obtaining additional patient flows to private clinics.

5. Elimination of barriers in terms of conditions and opportunities for providing paid services (their replacement by the provision of services by private organisations on the basis of the same institution).

The majority of state OBs face all sorts of (often unjustified) restrictions from higher authorities when organising the provision of paid medical services to the population for cash (while restrictions on the provision of paid services by cashless payment are established much less frequently).

Generally, these restrictions relate to the following:

- granting special authorisation to provide certain types of care on a paid basis. For example, very often the restrictions relate to the provision of medical care to children;
- restrictions on the distribution of income received from the provision of paid services: on the share of income from entrepreneurial activities allocated for labour remuneration; on the share of income (or labour remuneration fund) allocated for the remuneration of administrative and management personnel, etc.;
- opportunities for independent price setting, etc.

One form of a correct way out of such situations is the refusal of a medical institution to provide certain types of medical care on a fee-for-service basis, with the simultaneous provision of such an opportunity to a private HMO.

In fact, it is a matter of a private firm taking over the organisation of the provision of paid services. It uses the premises and equipment of a budgetary institution under certain conditions and engages employees of the budgetary institution. Accordingly, the private firm must reimburse the cost of the budgetary resources used, pay salaries to the engaged employees and incur other expenses out of the income received.

Naturally, for a budgetary institution this option is of interest, as a rule, only in a situation when it receives a part of the income received by a private organisation.

In many respects, this option of rendering paid services is more favourable for the state than the traditional mechanism of rendering paid services by budgetary institutions due to the following circumstances:

- private organisations, when providing services on the basis of the budget health care facility, pay rent, reimburse equipment depreciation, and utility payments. When providing paid services by the budget health care institution itself, reimbursement of budgetary resources used is not always ensured;

- there is no risk of unprofitability of entrepreneurial activity for the budgetary OZ;
- when conducting business activities by a private firm, there is always a lower level of shadow payment for medical services (due to stricter control, which is also facilitated by the smaller size of the private organisation, etc.);

Such advantages of private firms as higher flexibility, better organisation of the treatment process, economic and other aspects of the institution's activities, etc., (which in the end ensures higher efficiency), can become a good example and an object for study and copying by the budget institution.

In general, it can be concluded that the creation of a rational organisational and economic mechanism for the participation of private medical organisations in addressing public health issues is a rather complex problem.

However, the available, albeit small, experience of the Kyrgyz Republic demonstrates the possibility and necessity of strengthening public-private co-operation in the health sector, as will be discussed below.

In conclusion of this chapter, the following conclusions can be drawn from the problems of interaction between public and private health care that have been considered, far from being complete:

1. Legal mutually beneficial forms of cooperation between budgetary and private medical organisations are clearly underused.
2. Support for private health care should include aspects such as:
   - improvement of the legislative framework;
   - promoting the development of voluntary health insurance;
   - abandoning the policy of implicit discrimination against private medical clinics;
   - a more flexible pricing policy that ensures that private medical organisations, when participating in the MHI system or implementing the state order, reimbursement of reasonable costs;
   - creation of a clearer economic mechanism for the functioning of budgetary institutions, preventing the use of dumping prices when they provide paid medical services.

Chapter 4

Risk allocation in PPP project implementation

As noted earlier, the use of PPP mechanisms has firmly established itself in the world practice. Economic regional development is impossible without perfect transport, energy and social infrastructure, which, in turn, is possible only if there are extra-budgetary sources of financing. PPP mechanisms are used to attract private capital to create (modernise) and further manage public infrastructure.

Effective implementation of infrastructure projects in the regions requires a clear understanding of the principles of risk sharing, competence and responsibility of the parties involved.

It can be assumed that the main criteria for attributing this or that form of interaction between business and the state to public-private partnership are the level of risk transfer to the business sector, ownership rights to the constructed object, the terms of the contract for the right to receive income from the project [11, 14].

The most problematic criterion among those listed above is the transfer of risk to any of the project participants.

The matrix of distribution of different types of risk among PPP project participants is presented below (see table).

Table. Matrix of risk distribution between participants of regional infrastructure projects using the mechanism of public-private partnership

Types of risks	Risk allocation		
	Private sector	Private sector and the state	State
Design errors	v		
Provision of land			v
Obtaining licences, permits	v		
Risks of construction	v		

Hidden obstacles		v	
Commissioning	v		
Risks of exploitation	v		
Legislative changes, political risks			v
Currency and inflation risks		v	

Source: Sinyakova A.F., 2007.

As the authors correctly point out, when analysing the data in the table, it can be concluded that most of the risks, namely about 55.6 % are transferred to the private sector, another about 22.2 % lie entirely on the state and the remaining 22.2 % lie on the private sector and the state in equal proportions [14].

The main characteristics of regional infrastructure projects using PPP mechanism are the following:

1. A co-operation in which the private sector typically undertakes the design, construction, financing, utilisation and management of an asset, and then ensuring that the service is delivered to the public through the government or directly. The involvement of business in all stages is critical, and this is what distinguishes public-private partnerships from all previous forms of business-government interaction, where private business was only involved in the process of financing the project or only in the process of building and using the facility.
2. Revenue generation by the private sector, either through the collection of service user fees from the public or the government, or both.
3. Determination of the quality and quantity of the service provided by the state. If the state is responsible for the payment of user fees by the public, the state can adjust the fees depending on whether the service provided meets all the initial specifications of the project.
4. The level of risk transfer to the private sector is sufficient to ensure efficient project implementation. At the end of the contract, the government may own the asset created after paying a predetermined residual value to the private sector. The fair residual value depends on many market factors, and the risk of

impairment is borne by the government in this case.

Separately, it is worth considering the situation when PPP participants conduct their policies only with their own interests in mind (so-called behavioural risks). This often leads to the emergence of unplanned risks, which a priori lead to unaccounted costs associated with the design, financing, construction, operation, execution and drafting of contracts and other documents related to the project, monitoring and securing the partnership agreement. The main reason for such problems may be a divergence in the objectives of the partnership for the government and business. It should be borne in mind that the effectiveness of the partnership depends to a large extent on the behaviour of the private partners. Random factors as well as uncertainties in political, social, technological and economic conditions can contribute to diverging objectives.

Risks may manifest themselves at different stages of project execution depending on the nature and degree of influence of random factors in these stages.

Taking into account the range of potential PPP risks that partners may face, the risks and disadvantages of this form of co-operation are grouped into three main groups:

1. Economic, financial and currency risks, i.e. related to changes in exchange rates, inflation rate, economic growth rate, even purchasing power of the population, etc.

2. Technical (technological) risks, which are related to the process of construction, operation and maintenance of the partnership object.

3. Legal and political risks, which are related to changes in the political situation in the country, legislative framework, etc.

Chapter 5

Practical experience of Kyrgyzstan in the implementation of PPP projects.

The Kyrgyz Republic is taking initial steps to develop the PPP institute taking into account the best international practices.

As is well known, PPPs have been recognised worldwide as an alternative method to deliver public services and improve infrastructure facilities in a more efficient and quality manner.

PPP is an important direction of the state strategy for the development of the private sector in the country, which is confirmed by the adoption of the Law "On Public-Private Partnership in the Kyrgyz Republic" in 2012 [7], the programme for the development of public-private partnership for 2016-2021, approved by Government Resolution No. 327 of 16 June 2016, as well as the investment programme in the health sector for 2016-2025, approved by Government Resolution No. 359 of 30 June 2016. Thus, the PPP institutional framework was established and authorised state bodies were identified.

The process of preparation of the first PPP projects, including preparation of feasibility studies (hereinafter - feasibility studies) for further preparation for selection of private partners has been started. For this purpose, with the support of the Asian Development Bank, criteria for selection of PPP projects have been developed, approved by the Resolution of the Government of the Kyrgyz Republic "On financing the preparation of public-private partnership projects" dated 17 March 2014 No. 147, which establishes a transparent and balanced procedure for the preparation of PPP projects.

The Ministry of Health of the Kyrgyz Republic has initiated the development of the following PPP projects:

1. "Installation of computer tomographs in medical and preventive health care organisations of the Kyrgyz Republic on the terms of public-private partnership";
2. "Organisation of haemodialysis services in the cities of Bishkek, Osh and Jalal-Abad";
3. "Organisation of a centralised laboratory in Bishkek";
4. "Establishment and management of angiographic centres".

It should be noted that the above PPP projects are at different stages of implementation.

1. **PPP project "Installation of computer tomographs in medical and preventive health care organisations of the Kyrgyz Republic on the terms of public-private partnership".**

Project goal: to establish CT diagnostic centres in 10 health care institutions (2 in Bishkek, 8 in the regions).

Progress of PPP project execution.

This project was approved by the Supervisory Board of the PPP Project Preparation Financing Facility (PPPF) to finance the development of the project feasibility study (October, 2014).

On 1 July 2016, a contract was signed with the winning company (Rebel Group International BV, an international consulting company) and an agreement was concluded for the preparation of a feasibility study (hereinafter referred to as the Feasibility Study) and provision of transaction services (No. ADB-PPP-1).

In order to effectively implement the PPP project on the preparation of feasibility study, the order of the Ministry of Health of the Kyrgyz Republic "On the establishment of a working group for the implementation of the project on "Installation of computed tomography scanners in medical and preventive health care organisations of the Kyrgyz Republic on the terms of public-private partnership" dated 15 May 2017 № 396 was prepared.

The consulting company Rebel Group International BV submitted an Initial Report for the PPP Project for review and agreement in May. The Final Feasibility Study will be submitted in October 2017.

2. **PPP project "Organisation of haemodialysis services in Bishkek, Osh and Jalal-Abad" with grant support from the German Development Bank (KfW).**

Project objective: reorganisation and consolidation of haemodialysis services in 4 existing state haemodialysis units (2 in Bishkek, 1 in Osh, 1 in Jalal-Abad).

The Ministry of Economy of the Kyrgyz Republic approved this Draft Feasibility Study by Order No. 236-A dated 29 August 2016.

The tender documents were approved by the Order of the Ministry of Finance of the Kyrgyz Republic No. 206-P dated 22 December 2016.

The tender for the selection of the private partner was announced on 10 January 2017.

Applications for prequalification for the above project were received from the following 5 bidders within the deadlines set out in the Invitation to Tender and the PPP Project Tender Rules:

1) Nephrocare Health Services Private Limited (India)

2) TOO "Zhasandy Buirek" (Republic of Kazakhstan)

3) ESS GmbH (Germany)

4) Unit-Reactiv-Pharma LLC (Kyrgyz Republic)

5) Fresenius Medical Care Care Deutschland GmbH (Germany).

On 16 February 2017, a meeting of the tender committee was held to carry out a pre-qualification evaluation of the bids received.

Based on the results of the evaluation, two companies were selected and notified to send technical and financial proposals for the project to the tender commission within the established deadlines.

On 16 March 2017, an investor conference was held for companies that successfully went through the PPP project prequalification process.

The purpose of the conference was to discuss the provisions of the PPP Agreement between public and private partners, to agree on amendments and additions to the draft Agreement. Taking into account the discussions and comments received from the bidders, the draft Agreement was finalised and approved by the tender commission.

(PPP Agreement - a written contract between public and private partners defining the rights, obligations and responsibilities of the parties, other terms and conditions of PPP project implementation for the purpose of implementation of certain activities in various areas on PPP principles in the manner and forms established by the current legislation of the Kyrgyz Republic).

On 5 April 2017, the draft Agreement was sent to the Ministry of Finance of the KR for approval, in accordance with the PPP Law of the KR.

The draft Agreement was approved by the order of the Ministry of Health of the KR "On approval of amendments to the draft Agreement on the public-private partnership project "Organisation of haemodialysis services in the cities of Bishkek, Osh and Jalal-Abad" dated 19.04.2017 No. 232 and the order of the Ministry of Finance of the KR dated 20.04.2017 No. 62 - P.

The approved draft PPP Agreement was made available to bidders on 24 April 2017, with the bid submission date set for 26 May 2017. On 26 May 2017, technical and financial proposals from two pre-qualified companies were submitted.

On 14 June 2017, based on the results of the tender committee's evaluation, the winner was announced as Fresenius Medical Care, whose technical proposal was found to meet all requirements.

In accordance with the Law of the Kyrgyz Republic "On Public-Private Partnership in the Kyrgyz Republic", the public partner, represented by the Ministry of Health of the Kyrgyz Republic, proceeds to negotiations for further signing of the PPP Agreement with the winner of the tender.

In order to further effective implementation of the public-private partnership project "Organisation of haemodialysis services in Bishkek, Osh and Jalal-Abad", and in accordance with Article 18, paragraph 4 and Article 21 of the Law of the Kyrgyz Republic "On Public-Private Partnership in the Kyrgyz Republic from 22 February 2012 № 7, the Ministry of Health of the Kyrgyz Republic has prepared an instruction "On creation of an interdepartmental working group for technical support of the negotiation process between the state partner and the company - the winner of the tender, to sign a contract with the Ministry of Health of the Kyrgyz Republic".

The finalised draft PPP Agreement, taking into account discussions and additions received during the negotiation process with the private partner, the winner of the tender, was approved by the order of the Ministry of Health of the KR "On approval of the draft Agreement on the PPP project "Organisation of haemodialysis services in the cities of Bishkek, Osh and Jalal-Abad" dated 21.07.2017 No. 655. The Agreement on this PPP project was sent to the Ministry of Finance of the Kyrgyz Republic for approval.

The Ministry of Finance of the Kyrgyz Republic approved the draft PPP Agreement by Order No. 110-P dated 14 August 2017.

Key issues for PPP project implementation:

It should be noted that in order to conclude the PPP Agreement with the winning company and for successful implementation of this PPP project, an additional budget increase of 115.0 million KGS will be required (for the subsequent period starting from 2018).

At the same time, the cost of haemodialysis service provided by the private partner will include training of medical staff, service and maintenance of equipment.

As one of the options to resolve the issue - Providing tax relief or preferences:

> Article 12 of the PPP Law provides for the possibility of granting tax exemptions in accordance with the procedure and under the conditions stipulated by the KR legislation;

> According to Article 256-1 of the Tax Code of the Kyrgyz Republic, supply of services performed by a private partner in the process of implementation of a PPP Agreement is a supply exempt from VAT for the period set out in the PPP Agreement, **subject to the approval of the PPP Agreement by the Government of the Kyrgyz Republic.**

In connection with the above, a letter was prepared to the Head of the KR Government Office (copies - to all interested ministries and departments) regarding the exemption from VAT of services provided by a private partner under the PPP Agreement for the PPP project "Organisation of haemodialysis services in Bishkek, Osh and Jalal-Abad" and the need to prepare an order of the KR Government. In addition, a draft order of the Government of the Kyrgyz Republic was prepared, as well as a reference substantiation to the draft order of the Government of the Kyrgyz Republic.

The draft order of the KR Government on VAT exemption of services provided by a private partner under the PPP project "Organisation of haemodialysis services in the cities of Bishkek, Osh and Jalal-Abad" was approved by the Prime Minister of the KR dated 14 August 2017 No. 338-r.

On 15 August 2017, the signing ceremony of the PPP Agreement on the PPP project "Organisation of haemodialysis services in the cities of Bishkek, Osh and Jalal-Abad" was held between the Ministry of Health of the Kyrgyz Republic and Fresenius

Medical Care Care Deutschland GmbH (Germany).

3. **PPP project "Organisation of centralised laboratory in Bishkek".**

Project objective: organisation of a centralised laboratory in Bishkek.

The preliminary LLP version of the PPP project has been prepared and after going through the procedure of internal discussion with IFC management (International Finance Corporation), was submitted for review to the Ministry of Health of the Kyrgyz Republic on 22 December 2016.

In accordance with Article 16, Part 3 of the Law of the Kyrgyz Republic "On Public-Private Partnership in the Kyrgyz Republic" The feasibility study of the PPP project was also sent to the authorised state body in the field of PPP (Ministry of Economy of the Kyrgyz Republic) for discussion and decision making on further implementation of the above project (Annex: Feasibility Study on 412 pages).

Preliminary analysis of the Feasibility Study has shown that for successful implementation of the PPP project, additional financing from the state, to fulfil obligations to the private partner, in the amount of USD 2.5 million is required.

On 13.01.2017, an interdepartmental meeting was held to discuss the PPP project "Organisation of a centralised laboratory in Bishkek city", related to the problems of financing this project, identified by the results of the feasibility study.

In the period from February to April 2017, additional research was conducted to study the issue related to minimising the financial gap on the obligations of the public partner in financing the services of the private operator under the PPP project, various options were considered in terms of the volume of laboratory services provided in the context of health care organisations located in the territory of Bishkek.

On 20 April 2017, at the working meeting of the Ministry of Health of the Kyrgyz Republic and the Ministry of Economy of the Kyrgyz Republic on the implementation of PPP projects, it was decided that it was necessary to prepare an analytical note on the need to minimise the financial gap between the obligations of the public partner to finance the services of the private operator under this PPP project.

Key issues for PPP project implementation:

- Seeking funds to cover the financial gap between the current budget and funds required for PPPs (including taking into account possible receipt of funds from

ADB, within the framework of the Programme for Improvement of Investment Climate in the Kyrgyz Republic);

> Providing space for a central laboratory will help improve the attractiveness of the project to private investors;

> Tax exemptions or preferences (similar to the **PPP Project for organising haemodialysis services)**.

The issue of co-financing PPP projects on the establishment of dialysis centres and centralised laboratory was put on the agenda of the meeting of the Public-Private Partnership Council in the Kyrgyz Republic.

A meeting of the Council for Public Private Partnership in the Kyrgyz Republic was held on 16 June 2017

At this meeting it was decided to finalise the justification for the allocation of additional funding for the above projects with a focus on the economic component of the projects.

By decision of the Council for Public-Private Partnership in the Kyrgyz Republic, the Ministry of Finance of the Kyrgyz Republic conducted an additional analysis of the Feasibility Study to identify alternative sources of financing for the PPP project.

4. PPP project "Establishment and Management of Angiographic Centres".

Project objective: installation of an angiographic complex in a health care organisation and ensuring accessibility of the population to angiographic methods of diagnostics and treatment.

A tender for consulting services was announced. On 23 September 2016, the Tender Commission approved a short list of companies for further participation in the tender.

Technical and financial proposals were received from two companies within the deadline:

1) Consortium "Sanigest International", Central Asian Consulting Company "CAIConsulting" (Kyrgyzstan);

2) Grand Thornton Consortium (Armenia).

A Combined Technical and Financial Consultant Evaluation Report was prepared on 7 February 2017.

Based on the results of the evaluation of proposals, the tender commission recommended a re-tender with revision of the terms of reference and scope of work, due to a significant excess of the budget by $58,000. THE TENDER COMMISSION RECOMMENDED RE-TENDERING WITH REVISION OF THE TERMS OF REFERENCE AND SCOPE OF WORKS DUE TO SIGNIFICANT OVERRUN OF THE BUDGET BY USD 58 THOUSAND.

The required package of documents was prepared and submitted for approval to the Department of Public Procurement under the Ministry of Finance of the KR. On 10 July 2017, a repeated Request for Expression of Interest for consulting services to the Ministry of Health of the Kyrgyz Republic on this project was published on the website of the Ministry of Health of the Kyrgyz Republic and the Ministry of Economy of the Kyrgyz Republic.

A total of 8 companies submitted expressions of interest:

1. Inha University Hospital (South Korea);
2. TRANSPROEKT Group JSC (Russia);
3. management4health GmbH (Germany) / Avanco (KR);
4. BDO Unicon JSC (Russia);
5. Aninver InfraPPPP Partners S.L (Spain);
6. Grant Thornton Armenia (Armenia)/Grant Thornton Kyrgyzstan (KR);
7. Business quasar LLP (Kazakhstan);
8. Concept Realisation (UAE), HK Advisory (UAE), and GRATA International (KR).

On 14 August 2017, the collection of applications received was completed and companies were identified for shortlisting.

All eight companies that were sent a request for proposals for consulting services for the said PPP project on 5 September 2017 were shortlisted.

Chapter 6

Conclusion

The existing problems in the development of PPPs require the development of consistent steps for their successful resolution.

In order to eliminate the existing negative phenomena in the implementation of partnership relations between the state and private business, the following measures should be taken:

- Improvement, introduction of necessary amendments and additions to the current PPP legislation taking into account the practical experience of pilot projects implementation,
- preparation of methodological guidelines explaining the procedure of use of PPP principles;
- ensuring a fair distribution of opportunities and risks between government and private business (project risks should be borne by the partner that is best able to control and manage them; at the same time, it is irrational to shift all risks to the private partner, especially those risks directly affected by public policy);
- taking additional measures for transparent and efficient distribution of public contracts by creating competition for the right to implement the project;
- as part of the project feasibility analysis, it is crucial to develop realistic scenarios for forthcoming financing, which will enable an assessment of whether the project has sufficient potential to cover investment costs at current market rates over the life of the project;
- Amendments to the current tax legislation (introduction of a norm reflecting the specificity of PPPs in order to prevent problems related to increasing the tax burden of private investors without taking into account government intervention);
- compulsory risk insurance;
- Creating a favourable image of PPPs.

The existing experience of PPP creation and operation shows that one of the most important factors in ensuring the development of partnership relations between business and the state is a stable political environment and support for partnership. At the same time, an equally important role is assigned to the political and legal environment, which creates stable basic conditions for the development and implementation of PPP projects.

In conclusion, I would like to emphasise once again that the health care projects are the very first PPP projects in Kyrgyzstan implemented under the current legislation, and their successful implementation should serve as an example for attracting private sector and investment for further development, including the public health care system.

Investments in healthcare are characterised by a large multiplier effect. Together with economic feasibility, the implementation of PPP projects in the social sphere will significantly improve the quality of life of citizens. The healthcare sector, in addition to structural reforms, requires significant technological modernisation, which, in turn, requires serious investments.

Public funding for this sector, despite some growth, is still insufficient to have an impact on reducing mortality and increasing life expectancy.

Needless to say that establishment of fruitful co-operation with all stakeholders, exchange of opinions, experience and proposals for improvement of PPP activities, aimed ultimately at achieving the main goal - preservation and improvement of health of our citizens, improvement of quality of life - is one of the main levers in the development and establishment of PPP institute in the Republic.

Literature:

1. Database on Private Sector Participation in Infrastructure Projects. World Bank Group, www. woridbank. org.
2. Varnavskiy, V.G. Partnership of the state and private sector: theory and practice / V.G. Varnavskiy // World Economy and International Relations. - M., 2002. - №7. - C. 30 - 30.
3. Varnavsky V.G. Partnership of the State and Private Sector: Forms, Projects, Risks. - M., 2005. - C. 10 - 27.
4. In a crooked mirror (The OMC system, conceived as an analogue of the European social medical insurance, in fact turned into a variant of budget financing of state medical institutions) / Expert-North-West. - 2006. - № 23. - C. 33 - 36 // http://www.rosmedstrah.ru/articles.php?show=1&id=482&srch=1.
5. Gladkov, K.V. Public-private partnership as a source of competences of a private partner in healthcare / Modern problems of science and education. - 2016. - No. 2 // URL: http://www.science-education.ru/en/article/view?id=24359.
6. Derbina E.S. Prospects for the implementation of public-private partnership in the field of public health in the Russian Federation // Young Scientist. - 2014. - №17. - C. 259 - 261.
7. Law of the Kyrgyz Republic "On Public-Private Partnership in the Kyrgyz Republic" dated 22 February 2012 No. 7.
8. Constitution of the Kyrgyz Republic. Adopted by referendum (by popular vote) on 27 June 2010.
9. Makarov I.N., Kolesnikov V.V. National infrastructure and public-private partnership : the needs of the modern economics // Creative Economy. - 2012. - № 5 (65). - C. 50 - 54.
10. Mataev T.M. Prospects for the development of public-private partnership in the Republic of Kazakhstan // Russian entrepreneurship. - 2011. - No. 12, Issue. 2 (198). - C. 187 - 192 / http://www.creativeconomy.ru/articles/16129/.

11. National Report "Business Risks in the Private Sector". State Partnership" / Association of Managers. - M., 2007 // http://europeandcis. undp .org/uploads/public/file/PPPP%20Report 2007.

12. Practical Guide to Good Governance in Public-Private Partnerships / European Union economic commission. - New York - Geneva: UN, 2008. - 114 c.

13. Ranjith Appuhami, Sujatha Perera & Hector Perera. Management Controls in Public-Private Partnerships: An Analytical Framework. - Australian Accounting Review. - 2011. - No. 56, Vol. 21. - Issue 1.

14. Rastvortseva S.N., Fedyuk E.F. Distribution of risks between the participants of the public-private partnership projects . http://www.sworld.com.ua/index.php/ru/economy-411/business-economics-and-production-management-411/11274-411-0642.

15. Sinyakova A.F. Concession agreements: attraction of investments into the region by means of public-private partnership. - Regional economy: theory and practice. - M., 2007. - №10. - C. 59 - 64.

16. Soldatenkov V.Y. Concession as a form of public-private partnership: social aspect // Russian entrepreneurship. - 2010. - No. 6, Issue. 2 (161). - C. 46 - 50.

17. Financing the creation and modernisation of infrastructure facilities of transport and public utilities / Edited by J. Perrault, G. Chateloux. - Paris: Izd. of the French National Institute of Bridges and Roads, 2002.

18. Scherbuk, Yu.A.; Kadyrov, F.N.; Khairullina, I.S. Problems of interaction between public and private health care (in Russian) // Health care manager. 2008. -№ 2 / https://www.lawmix.ru/medlaw/10126.

Appendix

Reference on PPP project: "Organisation of haemodialysis centres in cities Bishkek, Osh and Jalal-Abad"

1	Name of public partner **Ministry of Health of the Kyrgyz Republic (hereinafter referred to as "M3 KR");**	
2	Project Name: **Organisation of haemodialysis centres in Bishkek, Osh and Jalal-Abad cities**	
3	General information about Project	M3 KR with the support of the International Finance Corporation (hereinafter - "IFC") and a group of consultants including Rebel Group International, Hogan Lovells (CIS) and Kalikova & Associates, are preparing a public-private project partnership (hereinafter referred to as "PPP") for the establishment of haemodialysis centres (hereinafter referred to as "the Project"). The Project is implemented with the financial support of the German development bank KfW. The project is designed to treat patients with chronic renal insufficiency provides for the reorganisation and consolidation of haemodialysis services in four existing national units haemodialysis in Bishkek, one unit in Osh and one unit in Jalal-Abad. It is envisaged to hold a tender for two lots [Lot 1: 1 haemodialysis unit in Bishkek + 1 haemodialysis unit in Jalal-Abad; Lot 2: 1 haemodialysis unit in Bishkek + 1 haemodialysis unit in Osh] and to conclude PPP agreements
4	Justification of the feasibility of PPPc application to the selected infrastructure	In order to justify the feasibility of PPP for the Project implementation, it should be noted first of all that in the field of haemodialysis the state faces certain difficulties, such as: lack of current capacity (financial and technical) to provide haemodialysis services to patients in need, lack

	facility. Justification that the PPP Project is in the interest of the State	of clear criteria to guide the M3 KR in selecting patients to receive haemodialysis services, etc. The project will be implemented by the Ministry of Health of the Kyrgyz Republic. Currently, there are about 1,300 patients in the KR with a
		different stages of renal failure, 709 patients require haemodialysis. Of this number, haemodialysis for 552 patients is financed from the state budget, since May 2016 the treatment of 118 patients is partially paid for from the Compulsory Medical Insurance Fund (from the total cost of 5500-6000 soms per procedure, 4900 soms is paid by the MHIF), 39 patients pay for the procedure themselves. However, it should be noted that these figures reflect only patients who have officially applied to the state for support. It is expected that the improvement of the haemodialysis service delivery system will be possible through the implementation of the Project through PPP. The PPP model to be implemented will cover four public centres in Bishkek, one centre in Osh and one centre in Jalal-Abad. The project will include 283 budget patients currently receiving haemodialysis services and will be able to offer better value for money. Better quality of haemodialysis services will be ensured, with some of the risks transferred to the private partner and at a price affordable to the government. In implementing the Project through PPP, there is a likely increase in patient coverage if the private company offers a lower than anticipated price, which will allow for an increase in the number of patients within the existing budget allocated to haemodialysis. The private partner is expected to improve the efficiency

		of haemodialysis service delivery (including management issues, premises, equipment and methodology) and to provide services to a higher standard than the existing ones. It is expected that the cost of providing haemodialysis services by the private partner will be lower than the cost of services currently procured by M3 KR from private organisations (SURFA)
5	Expected results from the Project implementation	Among the expected results from the Project implementation are the following: 1. Possible increase in patient coverage in haemodialysis centres; 2. The private partner is expected to provide services to higher quality standards than the
		the existing system in the KR; 3. The cost of haemodialysis services will be lower than the current cost paid under the M3 CD service contract with SURFA; 4. Improving the efficiency of the services provided (including, inter alia, management issues , premises, equipment, methodologies, etc.) 5. M3 The CD will bear significantly lower risks in the provision of haemodialysis services under the PPP model, the main risks will be on the private partner (e.g. equipment for the haemodialysis procedure is selected , is purchased and maintained by the private partner itself, quality standards for haemodialysis services must be adhered to by the private partner, etc.).
6	Strategic programmes (concepts)	- Programme on Transition of the Kyrgyz Republic to Sustainable Development of the Kyrgyz Republic for

	that include the Project	2013-2017 (approved by Resolution of the Government of the Kyrgyz Republic No. 218 of 30 April 2013); - Strategy for Protection and Promotion of Public Health of the Kyrgyz Republic until 2020 ("Health 2020") (approved by Resolution of the Government of the Kyrgyz Republic No. 306 dated 4 June 2014); - The National Programme for Reforming the Health Care System of the Kyrgyz Republic "Den Sooluk" for 2012-2016 (approved by Resolution of the Government of the Kyrgyz Republic No. 309 of 24 May 2012); - Healthcare Investment Programme for 2016-2025 (approved by Resolution of the Government of the Kyrgyz Republic No. 359 dated 30 June 2016)
7	Expected participation of organisations other than the state partner (Joint Stock Companies with state share, state-owned enterprise, institution or other economic entity).	On the side of the public partner in the PPP Project is the M3 KR. Funds for haemodialysis services will be accumulated in the payer's account for the services.
8	Location of the Project	Hemodialysis centres will operate in Bishkek, Osh and Jalal-Abad. The exact location of the Project has not yet been determined. One of the conditions of the M3 CD is that the private partner rents its own premises to carry out Project activities
9	Cost of feasibility study preparation	The German Development Bank (KfW) provided a grant for feasibility study preparation. Feasibility studies for haemodialysis centres include technical, legal and financial expertise. Total cost of feasibility study and tender for two PPP projects: (1) establishment of haemodialysis centres, (2) establishment of centralised of laboratories realised by the M3 CD is

		640,468 Euros
10	Preliminary assessment the total amount of capital investment required	Preliminary estimate of capital investment for one centre with 27 beds for hemodialysis services is: US$ 1.04 million. Capital expenditure is expected to be incurred on haemodialysis systems, processing units and water treatment systems, as follows: (i) Purchase of 27 units (24 units and 3 units). spare machine) for one haemodialysis centre. The cost of 1 machine is $17,000. THE COST OF 1 UNIT IS $17,000; (ii) Dialysis Chairs. Cost of dialysis chairs The cost of the armchairs shall be $2,200 each. The cost of each seat is US$ 2,200; (iii) If you choose to reuse dialysis machines, additional equipment must be purchased: - 2 dialyser re-treatment machines (cost is $5,650 each); - 1 re-processing operator and consumables sterilisation materials; (iv) Double reverse osmosis system (estimated cost of $93,000). It is assumed that one haemodialysis centre with 27 units requires 413 m of space[2] The private partner is expected to rent and renovate the premises with a cash investment of $170 per square metre. The private partner is expected to rent the premises and renovate it with a cash investment of $170 per square metre. The centre is also in need of additional
		contingency and monitoring equipment, viz:

		- Non-medical equipment with a value of $50,000. US$50,000; - Medical equipment valued at $45,000. THE COST OF THE MEDICAL EQUIPMENT IS $45,000; - In the fifth year of operation, a reinvestment of $50,000 is assumed. US$ 50,000
11	Estimated project implementation period	The PPP agreement will be concluded between the public and private partner for 10 years. After analysis by the consultants, this project term is the most optimal and has the greatest impact on the cost per haemodialysis session, i.e. with a contract duration of 10 years, the estimated price per session is the lowest. Duration of the contract

	Duration of the contract			
	4 years	6 years old	8 years	**10 years**
Cost of one haemodialysis procedure (USD)	68.60	63.40	61.10	**59.80**

12	Calendar plan project realisation	**Project Implementation Calendar Plan** **ScheduleStep**
		Counsellors December 2015 identified and selected
		Feasibility study preparation of the project, the structure of the project, the rules January - July 2016

			Tendering and tender documentation
		Июль - August2016	Initiation of the M3 CR Project; approval of the Project DOE of the Kyrgyz Republic; approval of the rules of conduct
			Tender and tender documentation, formation of the Tender Commission of the M3 CD; approval of the tender documentation by the MF CD
		August - September 2016	Announcement of the tender in mass media, providing open access to the tender rules and tender documentation to potential investors
		October - November 2016	Collection of applications for participation in pre-selection, evaluation of submitted applications, sending invitations to participate in the selection stage of the tender winner; presentations and meetings with pre-selected tenderers
		December 2016	Submission of tender offers by private partners at the stage of selecting

			the winner of the tender
		January - February 2017	Selection of the winner of the tender; announcement of the winner of the tender in the media; negotiations; approval of the draft agreement by the MoF; conclusion of the PPP agreement with the private partner
		**This timetable is provided for information purposes. Actual timing may vary depending on, among other factors, the timing of data availability and governmental decision-making, market conditions and investor interest.*	
13	Cost Estimates for: 1) Exploitation; 2) facility maintenance.	Expenditure on a haemodialysis centre with 27 treatment beds: (a) fixed costs - $350,000 US $ 350,000/year; (б) variable costs - US$ 1.03 million/year. (b) variable costs - US$ 1.03 million/year. The maintenance of the apparatus is modelled as a maintenance contract of $1,700 per year per apparatus. The maintenance of the apparatus is modelled as a maintenance contract of $1,700 per year per apparatus. The estimated annual maintenance costs for other equipment are 5 per cent of the investment cost. In addition to the total direct costs (heating, electricity, salaries, etc.), additional cost elements are included in the estimate. Costs related to cleaning, marketing, etc. are estimated to be around $5,100 - $9,600 per year, depending on the size of the centre. Costs associated with cleaning, marketing, etc. are estimated to be around US$ 5,100 - US$ 9,600 per year depending on the size of the centre	
14	Anticipated reimbursement of	Reimbursement is anticipated to come from the State's existing	

	expenses from: 1) service user charges (if applicable); 2) State contributions (if applicable); 3) other source of return on investment	budget for hemodialysis services. The MoH guarantees a minimum number of budget patients referred to the private partner and a corresponding minimum annual income per patient.
15	Expected number service users. Expected tariff for services	Expected number of users (budget patients): 283.
		Cost per session depending on various factors such as dialysis machine reuse, length of contract, number of machines, patients, etc.: $60 - $70. COST PER SESSION, DEPENDING ON VARIOUS FACTORS SUCH AS REUSE OF THE DIALYSIS MACHINE, CONTRACT PERIOD, NUMBER OF MACHINES, PATIENTS, ETC.: $60 - $70
16	Anticipated need and types of economic and/or financial state support	M3 and the Kyrgyz Government will grant certain rights under the Project, namely: State financial support: - Guaranteed payments by M3 through the opening of an escrow account; - Partial coverage of currency risks included in the contract is provided by means of fee adjustments in case currency fluctuations go beyond certain specified parameters; - A guaranteed minimum amount of work expressed in the form of a set level of minimum annual income.

		State economic support: - A private partner may provide dialysis services to "private" self-pay patients (whether paid for out-of-pocket or from other sources), as long as it is not at the expense or detriment of budget patients; - Access to government assets at reduced rates (zero rate possible). Types of state financial and economic support may be changed/added by the parties when preparing a PPP agreement. The private partner will be provided with the following services State guarantees stipulated by the legislation of the Kyrgyz Republic. The terms and conditions of the above types of state support and guarantees will be defined by the parties in the PPP agreement
17	The need to acquire land and its possible cost	No
18	Assessment of adverse environmental impacts of the Project: types and their expected costs	The main waste streams in haemodialysis centres include dialyzers, systems and needles. All of these can be categorised as solid waste consumables. Once used, all of these streams pose a risk of contamination to both visitors and employees of the haemodialysis centre. The collection of waste streams is organised by a private partner. In most cases, the waste is collected at one central point within the haemodialysis centre and incinerated. Haemodialysis centres must comply with medical waste management regulations, guidelines for safe transport, sterilisation and disposal of medical waste, emergency response and infection control measures, which are approved

		by M3 orders and KP government regulations. The private partner is obligated to: - obtain a waste disposal permit (issued by SAEPF on an annual basis); - to make payments for waste disposal in the environment in the amount of 3.24 soms per equivalent tonne of pollutants. The Project recommends that the private partner should contract with a specialised organisation. organising the removal and subsequent disposal of waste to avoid the costs associated with obtaining permits for independent waste disposal
19	Social assessment issues that may arise as a result of the Project, including the anticipated costs of addressing them	The most important issues relating to labour and working conditions are threefold: - Occupational risks for personnel Dialysis units (infection risk and workplace safety, use of hazardous materials, compliance with fire safety requirements); - Possible staff reductions, which may occur because the private partner provides haemodialysis services to a higher quality standard with fewer staff.
		Labour legislation of the Kyrgyz Republic provides for severance pay in the amount of 2 to 4 monthly salaries in connection with dismissal
20	Preliminary risk assessment (specify 5 main risks)	1. Limited budgetary resources to pay for haemodialysis services and risks associated with short-term budget planning; 2. Risks of failure to obtain licence and permit documents;

		3. Possible liquidation/bankruptcy of the private sector partner; 4. Change of financing terms or renegotiation of the loan agreement by financial institutions; 5. Lack of experience in implementing PPP projects in the Kyrgyz Republic
21	Minimum Requirements for the Project	Under the Project, the main responsibilities of the private partner are as follows: - Provide and maintain premises or other facilities for the provision of haemodialysis services to agreed standards for the duration of the PPP agreement, including the following options: - Restoration and maintenance of the premises provided for the territory of these national hospitals; and/or - Provision and maintenance premises in agreed locations; and/or - Provision and maintenance of other types of facilities and infrastructure , designed to ensure access to haemodialysis services by people living in the regions (e.g., support for peritonial dialysis) - Provide adequate haemodialysis equipment to achieve agreed quality/standards and volume of haemodialysis services throughout the term of the Agreement - Provide haemodialysis services for patients in acute condition.

		- Establish and maintain appropriate staffing levels in line with haemodialysis service standards and patient volumes, and conduct staff training activities - Select treatments that best meet the needs of each individual patient - e.g. peritoneal dialysis, etc.
		Package/Contract 1 Covered budget patients: - Bishkek - about 100 patients; - Osh - about 40 patients. The total number of budget patients is about 140 Number of machines in the centre: - Bishkek - about 17 apparatuses; - Osh - about 6 apparatuses. Children included. **Package/Contract 2** Covered budget patients: - Bishkek - about 119 patients; - Jalalabad - about 24 patients. The total number of budget patients is about 143 Number of machines in the centre: - Bishkek - about 19 apparatuses; - Jalalabad - about 5 apparatuses. Children excluded.

About the authors

Batyraliev Talantbek Abdullaevich - Ministry of Health of the Kyrgyz Republic, Minister, Doctor of Medical Sciences, Professor.

Ismailov Mederbek Adyshevich - Ministry of Health

Kyrgyz Republic, Head of the Department of Strategic Planning and Health Policy Development.

Abilov Bolot Aripovich - consultant, Doctor of Medical Sciences, Professor.

Corresponding author's contact information:

Name: Abilov Bolot Aripovich Abilov

Place of work: Ministry of Health of the Kyrgyz Republic, Consultant

Address: 1 Togolok Moldo St., Bishkek, 720000, Kyrgyz Republic E-mail address: b_abilov@mz.med.kg; abibol@yandex.ru Working phone: + 996-312-621903

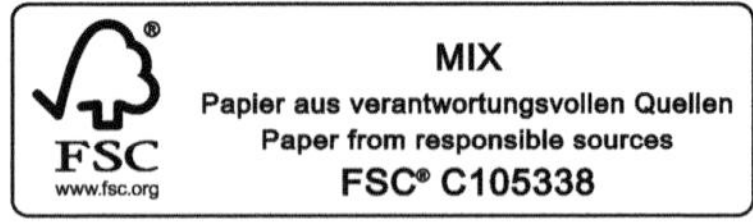

Printed by Books on Demand GmbH, Norderstedt / Germany